KRATOM

FOR PAIN RELIEF

TABLE OF CONTENTS

INTRODUCTION

Thank you for choosing *Kratom Book: "A Complete Beginner's Guide to Using Kratom Leaf – Kratom Teas, Kratom Extracts, Kratom Powders, and Kratom Capsules"* This book will educate you on everything you need to know about preparing and using Kratom Powders, Extracts, Tea and Capsule.

Kratom is a herbal supplement that has been used by South Asia Countries for centuries not only to improve mood and manage pain but also to increase stamina and energy levels, cure diarrhea and fight off fatigue among other benefits.

The Kratom leaf is a natural medication that was discovered in South East Asia. Many drug addicts across the globe are gradually reaching out to this herb as an alternative to stay out of heroin addiction. The leaf is understood to possess therapeutic properties apart from being stimulant and sedative in nature.

This guide is written to provide you with adequate information you need to start using kratom correctly to achieve the desired result. In this guide, you will also find information on various kratom strains and their effects, the legal stand of the herb, the recommended dose in grams and teaspoons, special precautions, possible side effects and more.

CHAPTER ONE

What is Kratom

Kratom is a tropical native tree of Papua New Guinea, Indonesia, Malaysia, and Thailand, where it leaf is being used for medicinal purposes because it has morphine-like effects. A large number of its health benefits are derived from the distinctive nutrients and chemical compounds discovered within the plant leaves, which include a variety of alkaloids and other organic materials that benefit various organs of the human body. The major active alkaloid in kratom which is also known as mitragynine is connected to being accountable for its opioid-like effects.

Kratom leaf is commonly chewed in the regions where the trees naturally grow, and it was estimated that about seventy percent of Thailand male population will chew about ten to sixty leaves in a day. They sell it as a leaf, capsule, gum, pellet, extract or powder, and it could be consumed as a tea, chewed or smoked.

The kratom tree's botanical name is Mitragyna speciosa. The history has revealed that it was banned in Thailand in the year 1979 (notwithstanding the fact that it's an indigenous product) as it was a regular substitute for opium, therefore affecting the country economy. Readily available for purchase kratom on the internet has come under the global limelight in recent years for its misuse as a recreational drug and its medicinal purpose. It was also banned in the country such as Myanmar, Malaysia, and Australia. In the European countries and the United State, Kratom is being progressively consumed by individuals withdrawing from opioid drugs like prescription painkillers and heroin or for the self-management of pain. Nevertheless, kratom usage is recommended in regions and countries where its distribution and possession are legally accepted.

CHAPTER TWO

Legal Stand of Kratom

Kratom legal position remains in a grey in America. The plant is officially legal on a federal level. Nevertheless, there are existing regulations for selling and using it in some states, while some other states have absolutely placed ban on it.

Here are the states that have imposed a ban and regulations on kratom:

- Alabama, the plant was marked in May 2016 as a schedule 1 controlled substance and was absolutely banned.

- Arkansas, the plant was also marked in February 2016 as a Schedule 1 controlled substance and was absolutely banned.

- California, the use of kratom was only banned in San Diego.

- Florida, the use of kratom was only banned in Sarasota County.

- Illinois, the law permits the sale of the drug to people above the age of 18 but was banned in Jerseyville.

- Indiana, the plant use has been absolutely banned.

- New Hampshire, the regulations only permit the kratom sales to people above the age of 18.

- Tennessee, the use of kratom has been absolutely banned.

- Wisconsin, the use of kratom has been absolutely banned.

There is still ongoing deliberation on whether kratom should be banned on a federal level or not. Many people are of the opinion that it should be banned since it possesses psychoactive properties which could turn into addictive. The opinion of others is that the plant may become an effective and efficient solution for dealing with the nation's opioid epidemic. For these motives, there are still lots of talk concerning the future legal stance of kratom.

In August 2016, the U.S Drug Enforcement Administration (DEA) decided to mark kratom as a Scheduled 1 controlled drug. This would place it on the same stand with Heroin, LSD, and Ecstasy. Though, the decision was reserved in October of the same year. Since then, nothing has been said by the Agency.

CHAPTER THREE

Health Benefits of Kratom

The leaf contains psychoactive opioid components that are similar to opiates and opioids. Taking the leaf will produce medicinal effects, such as relieving pain and uplifting moods. It is versatile, so could be used as an aphrodisiac and can treat a wide range of conditions and disorder. The common benefits of kratom include:

1. Pain Relief

The leaf of kratom has in analgesic properties and could rapidly relief pain all through the body by influencing the hormonal system. When the leaf is chewed, the volume of the dopamine and serotonin released into the body system increases. This consequently eases the pain. Basically, the alkaloids overcast the pain receptors through the entire body system. The opium-like or morphine value of kratom leaf is commonly regarded as its most important application.

2. Immune System Booster

Independent researches on the numerous alkaloids found in kratom leaf have revealed that the combined effects could have great impacts on the resilience and strength of the immune system. The leaf extracts of the kratom that were traditionally used as herbs, are a natural source of antioxidants and are blessed with antimicrobial activities and free radical scavenging.

3. Energy Booster

Part of the reasons why kratom leaf is well-liked, predominantly among manual workers in various countries is the metabolic effects it possesses. It can raise the level of your energy by impacting hormone levels and boosting certain metabolic processes. These are the results of improved circulation, notwithstanding its calming nature, combining with increased metabolic actions to supply a boost of energy and a general upsurge in oxygenated blood to the areas of the body where it is needed. Kratom leaf is often an alternative natural therapy for those suffering from Chronic Fatigue Syndrome.

16

4. Sexual Stimulant

Kratom leaf is perceived by most users and traditional physicians as a fertility booster and an aphrodisiac, as the flow of blood and extra energy could help revitalize a tired libido, increase fertility, and improve sexual desire.

5. Reduced Anxiety

The leaf of kratom is commonly used as anxiolytic components for those suffering from mood swing, anxiety, depression, and chronic stress. By way of regulating our body hormones, we could now be relieved from all these wearing symptoms of chemical inequity without depending on pharmaceutical medicines and all of their inherent side effects

6. Addiction Recovery

As a result of the intrinsically healthy nature of kratom leaf, coupled with its series of impacts, it has been used as a corrective therapy for addiction for hundreds of years. Addiction has been a major issue in many opium and cultures, chewing the leaf often provides alike sensation without the negative and comedown side effects. Consequently, when people are making efforts to get clean, they usually make use of kratom leaf as a bearable remedy, thus making the leaf very treasurable in many parts of the world. It also assists to cover departure symptoms in the transition, away from that extra powerful drug.

7. Diabetes Treatment

The impact of the kratom leaf on blood sugar levels is among its least recognized benefits. Various studies have revealed that the alkaloids discovered in the leaf are capable of regulating the amount of glucose and insulin in the blood, successfully averting the dangerous troughs and peaks that are encountered by diabetic's patients. This doesn't only assist diabetic in managing their condition, but also stop it from developing in the first place.

8. Enhance Sleep

Kratom is known for its ability to helps insomnia by stimulating sleep and also increases the intensity of sleep thus making you feel rejuvenated and refreshed every morning.

CHAPTER FOUR

Kratom Strains and Their Effects

There are several Kratom's (Mitragynine) strains. Every one of them provides distinct chemical properties that lead to specific curative effects. The following are the most prevalent strains:

- Bali, it provides euphoric effects and other effects alike to opioid usage.

- Green Vein Kali, it has a stimulating strain with painkilling components.

- Maeng Da, it provides an invigorating effect that also relieves aches.

- Red Vein Kali, it possesses a soothing effect such as opioids.

- Ultra Enhanced Indo is an extract with sturdy euphoric impacts.

- White Vein Kali, it possesses euphoric and disassociating impacts.

Apart from the extract, people would only need ½ to 3 tsp of the leaf to get the needed effect. A lesser to a gram amount of extracts would provide similar effects to that of leaves as they are more strong.

Kratom has been used to treat disorders, social anxiety, pain, and other condition for years. Just a little dose is required to get the desired results. This is the reason behind people's acceptance of the natural plant. It is versatile, affordable, and effective.

CHAPTER FIVE

Usage Methods

Kratom powdered leaf can be taken through several methods, prepare as a tea, mixing with food and, "toss and wash" are the most common among them. The below tips will assist users to choose the best method of taking kratom.

1. Prepare as a tea

It is effective and convenient. Keep in mind that you can only make tea with the powdered leaf, do no use extracts as the hot water might damage some of the alkaloids. Begin by measuring out one tsp of powdered leaf. Boil two cups of water. Plenty of water will reduce the toughness of the flavor but still, maintain the same effects.

Put the powder in a large container or cup. Pour the boiling water on it. Stir thoroughly using a spoon. You can add honey, artificial sweetener, or sugar to taste, and then stir. Allow it to cool for about 15 minutes. As soon as it is cooled, the powder will settle to the bottom of the container. You can now pour the tea into a small cup and drink. You can add ice cube or water to neutralize the flavor but still maintain the same effects.

I also recommend my favorite tea recipe for you: I suggest preparing this at night before bed. It would be ready for you in the morning.

Ingredients:

- One cup of water

- One chamomile tea bag

- One spearmint tea bag

- Two teaspoons kratom

- Artificial sweetener, honey or sugar to taste

- One teapot

Instructions:

- Boil water in a kettle.

- Place kratom with both teabags in the teapot and pour boiled water on top.

- Allow it steep for 20-30 minutes.

26

- Remove tea bags.

- Place teapot in the fridge and leave it overnight. Kratom would settle to the bottom.

- Carefully pour the tea into a cup in the morning. Ensure you stop pouring when you observed the plant substance is about coming out. Dispose of the settled kratom substance left in the teapot.

- Add sweetener and drink.

2. Mixing kratom with food

You can mix with your favorite recipes such as ice cream or applesauce. Mixing with chocolate protein powder or chocolate almond milk are other good suggestions. Remember that it possesses a strong flavor and might not combine well in some specific foods. Taking it with a small quantity of any of the suggested recipes or food would not lessen the kratom effectiveness.

3. Toss and wash

You only need to spoon the powdered leaf into your mouth and wash it down with fluid. This method is considered the most difficult but offers the strongest impacts. The powder is extremely dry and would stick to your mouth and throat, making users to cough it out of their mouth. The ideal thing is to spoon little amount at a time when using this method

4. Use in capsule form

You can capsule it yourself instead of buying the pills. This is surely a convenient method of using kratom without even having a bit of the taste. Nevertheless, the only issue with this method is that it requires a couple of capsules at a time to have an adequate dosage of kratom (10+pills). Use with sufficient water and you will be fine.

CHAPTER SIX

Dosage and Precautions

The kratom dosage to take depends on what experience you want to have. You can determine the usage whether for instant energy, mental clarity or pain relief. You can take it either measured in teaspoons or as grams. It's important to measure the kratom dosage correctly to avoid overdose and the hazard involved with it. An electronic weighing scale can be used to measure dose accurately.

1. Dosage in Gram

Just like using something new, you may experience symptoms such as headache or nausea before you get used to it. As soon as the feelings are gone, the dosage can be determined based on the form that you find convenient and the strain of the kratom.

- Dosage for Focus and Energy: 3-6 grams per day. Effects differ from individual to individual. To improve the effectiveness of the dosage, mix it with grapefruit juice.

- Dosage for Pain relief and Anxiety: 7-9 grams will give the needed results. It's ideal to gradually begin with smaller dosages because higher dosages produce sedating effects.

- Dosage for Opiate Withdrawal: There is the claim that kratom can completely withdraw opiates with measured doses which decrease in frequency. Start with 7-9 grams and take 3 or 4 times daily for the first 3 days. Reduce the dose to 5-7 grams on the fourth day. The fifth day, reduce it 3-5 grams and on the sixth day, take only 2 grams. You can stop taking Kratom from day 7 on.

2. Teaspoon Dosage

A teaspoon can also be used to measure the kratom powdered leaf dosage in the absence of an electronic scale. A teaspoon full powder contains about 4-5 grams, depending on the packaging and the texture of the powder. If you are a beginner, start with a low quantity. For energizing and mood elevation take 1 to 1½ teaspoon of powdered leaf per day to get better effects. Anything more than 9 grams in a day is dangerous to health.

3. Capsules Dosage

Some individuals have chosen buying capsules to avoid stress since measuring the precise dosage of the powdered leaf is very important. There are jumbo packs of capsules that contain 1000 mg of powdered leaf, but most capsules contain 500-600 mg. Therefore, clarify with the seller, the capsule size for you to decide the quantity to take.

Notes:

Do same for every new strain you attempt to use, for you to discover your needed dosage for a specific strain. It is ideal that you consume kratom on an empty stomach, hence take it first in the morning or two to three hours after the meal. Taking kratom with food in your stomach would require a higher dosage. So I recommend taking it first on an empty stomach for a start.

Precautions:

Here are a few things worthy of knowing when using kratom as a beginner, or you are trying a new strain you have never taken before.

- Remain hydrated: Kratom would dehydrate you quickly just like coffee, so be sure you drink plenty of water with it. If you have a slight feeling of "heady" that means you need to drink more water. Consequently, bear in mind that you will need more fluid than normal when using kratom.

- Take on an empty stomach. As I have mentioned before, this is very significant, particularly for new users. As time goes by you could try out using the powdered leaf with food in your stomach but the best thing is to have a reference point. Taking with a full stomach would require more dosage which will be accompanied by the side effects.

- Each strain might need a different dosage. Follow the above dose recommendations each

35

time you are trying a new strain. This is important as various strains might have different sweet spots for you. A number of the faster strains could certainly hit harder. This is why you need to start on a low dose for each strain.

- Keep a record. This will help to take notes of your first experience with each strain, including the time you used it, the quantity you used and more. Write down your feelings and thoughts as you have them. This would assist you in building on each of your experiences when you refer back to the record

CHAPTER SEVEN

Kratom Side Effects

Though kratom leaf does have various therapeutic effects, it does equally have some side effects. The dosage taken has great influence on the deepness of the side effect. Kratom consumers have more likelihood of experiencing side effects if taking average to high dosages that is from seven to fifteen grams. The length and the purity of the drug use would also determine whether the consumer will experience a side effect or not. While some side effects are moderately minor, some could be severe.

Common side effects include:

- Hyperpigmentation

- Nervousness

- Vomiting

- Tremors

- Agitation

- Aggression

- Constipation

- Delusions

- Hallucinations

- Nausea

- Respiratory depression

Long-term usage could also result in additional symptoms, such as constipation, anorexia, weight loss, and dry mouth. For these reasons, be cautious while using kratom for medical purposes. If any of these symptoms persist or aggravated, stop usage and consult your physician.

CHAPTER EIGHT

Is Kratom Addictive?

Use of kratom for long-term can result in both psychological and physical dependence. Research has revealed that more than 50 percent of those who consumed kratom frequently for six months developed addiction on the medicine. The reason for this is that kratom is an addictive material, and could possibly be abused.

Kratom is addictive due to the fact that it possesses chemical properties which are alike to opioids. The medicinal plant could stimulate opiate signaling and subsequent pathway in the brain. It implies that consumers of kratom would experience a strong and high exhilarated sensation. This is the way the plant treats opiate dependences and decreases their withdrawal symptoms intensity. The chemical composite essentially works similar to a less potent type of methadone and heroin. One of the major worrisome aspects of kratom leaf usage is that the body could develop tolerance. It implies that a bigger dose is required to have the same impact. Tolerance is the bases for users to develop obsessive drug seeking manners, and would also result in overdoses.

KRATOM ABUSE DETECTION METHODS:

Though kratom has properties similar to opioids, they are not related functionally. This implies that they cannot be detected via opiate drug tests. And it does not imply that its metabolites are not present in the consumer's body system. But it's just that ordinary drug test cannot detect its presence. Most usual drug test check for opiates, PCP, amphetamines, cocaine, and marijuana only. The meaning of this is that kratom would still not be detected in this test.

Fortunately, there are some kits and specialized drug tests that could discover the use of kratom. These discovery methods would require either a blood or urine sample. It takes at least five days for kratom alkaloids to totally go off the urine. Therefore, urine drug tests can detect the use of kratom for up to one week.

Blood tests search for Mitragynine concentrations. The concentrations have to surpass 300ng/ml for the test to be positive. Unluckily, Mitragynine and its metabolites can only be detected in the blood for the first 24 hours.

SYMPTOMS OF KRATOM ADDICTION WITHDRAWAL:

As much as most long-term kratom consumers would cultivate a physical dependence on it, they would experience withdrawal symptoms when they quit. The magnitude of the withdrawal symptoms will depend on the length and the dose of the drug that had been used.

Here are some of the common withdrawal symptoms:

- Runny noses

- Profuse sweating

- Panic attacks

- Nausea and vomiting

- Muscle and joint pain

- Mood swings

- Irritability

- Intense cravings

- Insomnia and sleep disorders

- High blood pressure

- Diarrhea

These withdrawal symptoms could be somewhat difficult to tolerate. It could be so deep that they result in relapses. Most people with addiction to kratom would need to seek professional advice to combat the symptoms.

KRATOM OVERDOSE SYMPTOMS

Too much of kratom dosage is what perhaps leads to an overdose. The drug's effects manifested immediately after it's being taken, and could stay for hours. That means the symptoms of overdose could stay longer.

Common symptoms of overdose include:

- Seizures and tremors

- Respiratory depression

- Paranoia

- Nausea and vomiting

- Lethargy

- Delusions

- Combative or aggressive behavior

Overdose users may possibly experience severe nausea. It may even result in hallucinations, confusion, and hostility in extreme situations.

KRATOM WITHDRAWAL TIMELINE

Kratom would normally remain in the bloodstream for about sixty to ninety minutes. Once the drug leaves the body, the withdrawal symptoms will start reflecting. It only takes a few hours in most cases. These symptoms often persist within two to three days. This is relatively similar to the opiate and opioid withdrawals timelines. During this period, kratom consumers find it difficult to concentrate, get goosebumps, and experience intense craving. Most of the symptoms of withdrawal would stay for about seven to ten days. At this point, the withdrawals come to be less physical than psychological. Until months later, the intense craving might not subside.

The withdrawal timeline varied from different individuals. This is apparently because each individual's body system responds to the drug differently. People that are less dependent on kratom often get milder symptoms. However, there are several other factors that determine the withdrawal timeline's length. Some of the most common factors include:

1. Co-occurring disorders

People having co-occurring disorders are more probable of having more intense withdrawal symptoms. There is also every possibility for the symptoms to often stay longer. It is important to treat both the disorder and addiction simultaneously.

2. Dosage Used

Higher doses result in longer withdrawal timelines.

3. Environment and support system

The quality of an individual's withdrawal can be affected by their various environments. A person withdrawing in a high-stress environment may experience more prolonged and severe withdrawal symptoms.

4. Genetics

The biological makeup of an individual will contribute to the metabolisms of the drug in the body. And also influence an individual's responsiveness to withdrawals. An individual's biological makeup can contribute to how the drug is metabolized. It also affects how a person will respond to withdrawals.

5. Length of drug use

The longer a person has been taking kratom, the more the probability of experiencing deep withdrawal symptoms.

6. Abuse Method

Snorting or smoking the leaf would have a stronger effect than drinking or chewing it. Combining kratom with alcohol and other drugs could also result in more severe withdrawal symptoms. The users are also most liable to more withdrawal symptoms. Alcohol and other drugs could easily make the impact of kratom usage more complicated.

Since stress can aggravate the symptoms of withdrawal, built-up addiction treatment has therefore been recommended by many experts when withdrawing from kratom usage. These treatment approaches are able to provide relaxed and peaceful atmospheres.

CHAPTER NINE

Important Tips for a Healthy Living

Physical fitness is not the only justification for being healthy, emotional and mental fitness also contributes to it. Being healthy should be part of your over-all way of life. Keeping a healthy lifestyle could assist in preventing long-term illnesses and chronic diseases. Taking care of your health and feeling good about yourself is essential for your self-image and self-esteem. Doing what is ideal for your body is maintaining healthy living. If you want to be a well-rounded healthy person, the following health tips will help you to be just that.

1. Maintain a Regular Routine Exercise

You don't have to force yourself into extreme aerobics at the gym but you have to stay as active as you can. You could stick to walking, Swimming, easy floor exercise, or simply keep yourself going by doing various household routines. Engage in what is allowed by your body to do. The most important thing is that you keep on exercising. Dedicate not less than 20 to 30 minutes daily to exercise for about 3 to 5 times weekly. Have a routine. Ensure you have sufficient physical activities on a daily basis.

2. Watch Your Diet

You need to keep eating healthy food to maintain a healthy lifestyle. Add more vegetables and fruits in your diet. Eat less unhealthy, high sodium fat, and carbohydrates. Avoid eating sweets and junk food. Avoid missing a meal as this would make your body desire extra food once you start eating. Think of burning more calories than you consume.

3. Surround Yourself with Positive Drive

For you to have a sound emotional and mental state, you ought to surround yourself with optimistic energy. You cannot avoid all life's obstacles, but it helps to approach such difficulties with a positive mindset. Surround yourself with good people and friends that would offer you constructive criticism from time to time to help you progress. Make it a practice to always see the brighter aspect of life. There is always an upside (something positive and good) to every worst situation.

4. Increase Your Water Consumption

When your primary objective is eating right and getting in shape, you may not give due priority to drinking sufficient water. As you are striving to maintain your healthy habits, nonetheless, it is essential to add to your water ingestion. Apart from keeping you hydrated and improving the functions of your body, water consumption will also help in maintaining your weight. Cultivate the habit of drinking a cup of water before every meal, and the feeling of richness you will have can help in reducing your calories intake.

5. Enjoy Yourself

For you to keep a healthy lifestyle you need to enjoy your life. Engage in activities that give you fun and happiness, and don't allow your age to take the life out of you. Don't get yourself too serious. Set aside time to catch fun if you are a workaholic, connect with people and laugh. Also ensure you set aside time each day for engaging in anything such as going to the cinema, taking a bubble bath, taking a walk, meditating, etc.

6. Get a Full Night Sleep

Life is full of commitment and activities, if you don't make time for sleep, your objective of keeping a healthy lifestyle can be jeopardized.

Not having enough sleep can result in problems with mood concentration, and focus fluctuation. Indeed, inadequate sleep brings about unhealthy decisions, as it lessens activities in the part of your brain that manages impulse control. Thus, try to get an average of 7 to 9 hours of sleep each night

7. Quit Smoking

Smoking does not only damage your organs, lungs, and overall health but also harmful and expensive to the people around you. For you to live as long as possible and maintain a healthy way of life, you may need to consider refraining from it if you are a habitual smoker.

8. Stay Mentally Inspired

To maintain a healthy living, never stop learning new things even if you have graduated from school. There are numerous affordable and convenient means for you to continue learning. Search for various online courses and enroll yourself. It's crucial to continuously set goals and challenge yourself.

9. Visit Your Doctor Regularly

Regular consultation to your doctor and dentist will make you ascertain you are on the right track to keeping a healthy lifestyle. You will observe that as you are getting older, you will start experiencing strange happenings in your body. As a result of this, it's significant to keep update with medical tests, checkup, and screening.

BENEFITS OF BEING HEALTHY

- Keep our mind Healthy and happy

- Prevent injury by strengthening our bones and muscles

- Upsurge energy by making food choices and healthy way of life.

- Prevent diseases like diabetes, strokes, and heart attacks

- Enjoy good mental health to fight against anxiety, depression, and also to strengthen our minds.

- Keep healthy weight that would help lessen the risk of stroke and increase the overall image of ourselves.

Keeping a healthy living is so simple, it does not require lots of effort, just continue doing what you do and put in the above keeping healthy tips – definitely, you would soon become a well-rounded healthy being.

www.ingramcontent.com/pod-product-compliance
Lightning Source LLC
Chambersburg PA
CBHW021256280526
45784CB00005B/2391